Reflux

— — — — — ❧❧❧❧ — — — — —

Finally free: Stop heartburn and excessive acid in less than a week with these natural methods along with a tasty diet.

Table of Contents

—————— ✤✤✤✤ ——————

Additionally, the information in the following pages is intended only for informational purposes and should thus be thought of as universal. As befitting its nature, it is presented without assurance regarding its prolonged validity or interim quality. Trademarks that are mentioned are done without written consent and can in no way be considered an endorsement from the trademark holder.

Introduction

⸺⸺⸺ ❧❦❧❦ ⸺⸺⸺

Congratulations on downloading this book and thank you for doing so.

The following chapters will discuss acid reflux, also known as heartburn or GERD, common symptoms, common treatments and natural solutions to try to relieve symptoms without medication.

The majority of our population has suffered from occasional symptoms of acid reflux within the last year. Those are some pretty strong statistics. If you or a loved one suffers from occasional heartburn or even persistent symptoms, this is for you.

Relieving symptoms of acid reflux seems like it would be easy. Most people think that reflux is simply caused by too much acid produced in the stomach. Unfortunately, that is only a small part of the problem, and trying to solve the problem using that logic leads to bigger problems. In the following pages, you will find a concise list of causes of acid reflux and GERD, ranging from the simple, "too much stomach acid" to the more complex issues of bacterial growth.

A review of home remedies, dietary and lifestyle changes, and prescription medication options will be discussed, as well as their benefits and side effects. You will also find a number of diet protocols including a 3-day sample meal plan for living with acid reflux symptoms.

This guide is meant to inform, and not to be used in replacement of medical advice. While there are certainly a number of remedies to try, it is important to consult with your

Introduction

doctor before beginning any new regimen. Your doctor review your medical history and will discuss the positives and negatives of the treatment you plan to try, and determine if the regimen is safe for you. It is important to report any side effects or adverse symptoms associated with any treatment, so that it may be addressed before any serious complications arise.

There are plenty of books on this subject on the market, thanks again for choosing this one! Every effort was made to ensure it is full of as much useful information as possible, please enjoy!

Chapter 1:
What is heartburn?

Acid reflux, or gastroesophageal reflux disease (GERD) is simply the presence of stomach acid in the esophagus. The acid, with an average pH of 2 is strong enough to irritate and damage the lining of the esophagus, causing a 'burning' sensation, commonly called 'heartburn'. This condition has several symptoms including:

- Burning and pain in the chest
- Sore throat
- Burping, taste of acid in throat
- Regurgitation of food and acid mixture in throat

How is GERD Diagnosed?

Occasional heartburn happens to just about everyone, but some suffer on a weekly, or even daily basis with symptoms. As this consistency develops, GERD can be diagnosed. In most cases, GERD is diagnosed based on the symptoms alone, but other tests are available to confirm a diagnosis. A 'barium swallow' is a type of x-ray done to the upper GI and chest region. The patient drinks a liquid that coats the lining of the esophagus and stomach. This allows the area to be seen on x-ray, helping the doctor determine if any damage has been done by continuous exposure to stomach acid. The barium swallow is perhaps the easiest way to diagnose GERD for the patient, as it is non-invasive.

The doctor may also choose to do a full endoscopy, a procedure in which a small tube with a camera on the end is inserted down the throat, taking video on the way down. This allows the doctor to pinpoint any damage that has occurred on video, a major step above looking at the area on an x-ray. The doctor looks for signs of inflammation and ulcers, and varying sizes of holes in the epithelial lining of the esophagus. This method is superior because less obvious scarring will show up more clearly than in a barium swallow, making a possible diagnosis of the problem much sooner. Often the patient is sedated for this procedure, as it is quite invasive and unpleasant for the patient.

During the endoscopy, the doctor may choose to set up a monitoring device to measure pH levels in your esophagus and stomach. A small device can be "clipped" to the lining of the esophagus, taking data for a couple of days before falling off. These devices are designed to pass through the GI system without causing any harm to the patient. Data collected over this time span can help the doctor determine specific times where acid reflux is worst. It can then be compared to food logs to help determine food triggers, both the type of food and the amount consumed. Once a diagnosis is made, a treatment plan can be put in place to relieve symptoms and decrease stress and damage in the esophagus.

What happens if acid reflux persists untreated?

If left untreated, persistent exposure of esophagus to acid can lead to permanent damage and scarring of the esophagus, called Barrett's Esophagus, or Barrett's syndrome. As the esophageal lining is exposed to more and more acid, the cells change to resemble a stronger, tougher intestinal lining that is able to handle the acid. A normal esophagus is made up of squamous cells, meaning flat and thin, and there is a transition to columnar epithelial cells, meaning tall and skinny, in the stomach, intestines and lower GI system. Endoscopy can detect this change in cells, indicating long-term damage caused by acid reflux.

Barrett's esophagus does not have any specific symptoms outside of acid reflux, but is a clear sign that GERD has remained consistent over a long period of time. According to WebMD, having a Barrett's diagnosis increases the risk of developing esophageal cancer, but is still rare, only occurring in about 1% of Barrett's sufferers. Once Barrett's syndrome has occurred, it is very unlikely that it can be reversed. Finding out the cause of the acid reflux that led to it may help relieve symptoms for the patient, but the scarring is most likely permanent.

Long term exposure to stomach acid also begins to form squamous cell carcinoma, a cancerous cell that can develop into masses, and can spread to other parts of the body. A person who is diagnosed with Barrett's esophagus will be closely monitored via endoscopy to determine if this condition is developing.

New treatments are becoming available in order to remove Barrett's tissue to prevent the formation of cancer. Ablasion through heat or freezing can eliminate questionable sections of tissue before given the chance to become cancerous. In cases where formation of cancer is imminent, the doctor may recommend full removal of parts of the esophagus that cause the most problems, called esophagectomy. Treatment like this is usually only done on young patients who will have more chance of developing cancerous cells in the esophagus over their lifetime than a person at the end stages of life would have.

Since none of these treatments seem that pleasant, it is important to see a doctor as soon as symptoms begin to develop a pattern, or are seen consistently. Early detection and prevention is the best method to avoid esophageal damage leading to more serious problems like Barrett's syndrome or cancer. Your doctor will only know you have an issue with stomach acid if you tell them, so do not hesitate to do so. There may be a simple solution to your problem that will eliminate symptoms and prevent damage in the future.

Why is stomach acid necessary anyway?

Stomach acid is one of the first substances, after saliva, to treat food entering the GI system. The primary function is to kill off potential pathogens before they are allowed to enter the bloodstream, potentially causing illness throughout the body. These gastric juices consist of natural hydrochloric acid produced by parietal cells in the stomach lining. This acid has a pH of about 2, similar in strength to battery acid. The stomach lining, where the acid originates, is made of columnar epithelial cells, which are designed to be able to handle the high acidity of gastric juice, causing little to no harm. A problem occurs when cells with less resistance to this acid are exposed, like the more delicate squamous cells of the esophagus.

Why does gastric juice need to be so acidic? The GI tract acts as the body's first line immune system defense against foreign invaders. All living beings are required to take in nutrients from their environment in order to survive. The problem is, other substances, like toxic chemicals or disease-causing bacteria and viruses often accompany food as it enters the body. As food, or other substances enter the body, the GI system separates food particles from potentially harmful toxins and bacteria. Once a toxin is isolated, the acid breaks through the offending cell's defenses and neutralizes it, protecting the body. The body's natural defense is normally enough to kill any invading bacteria. More acid resistant strains, like Salmonella or Shigella commonly cause food poisoning, regardless of the body's best defenses. Even though the body is able to take care of itself for the most part, it is important to thoroughly cook food to kill the majority of possible pathogens before they get in the body, lessening the chance of sickness.

Stomach acid also play a major role in the digestion of food, breaking it down into smaller, more usable forms of nutrients. Gastric juices break down food particles down into their basic nutrients, carbohydrates (sugars), amino acids (proteins) and lipids (fat). Carbohydrates make up familiar foods like pasta, rice, and bread. Amino acids are from proteins like beef, chicken, fish or plant-based beans and soy. Lipids are broken down from fats that exist in foods like meat, olive and coconut oil and dairy products. Without it, these macronutrients would fail to absorb into the bloodstream when they reach the small intestine, which would make them virtually useless to the body.

What happens if stomach acid is too low?

If stomach acid is too low and this part of the digestion process does not occur, malnutrition can develop, even though a good source of food is entering the body. The same goes for necessary vitamins and minerals. Without proper absorption, deficiencies can occur, leading to sickness in the body. A good example would be iron, a mineral usually found in meat products. It is better absorbed in the presence of acid, like citrus juices. With an absence of stomach acid to help absorb it, iron simply passes through the digestive system, and is excreted, unused by the body. Iron deficiency can present with symptoms of fatigue, and, if not addressed, can lead to neurological problems.

Chapter 2:
Possible causes of acid reflux

There is not one single cause of acid reflux, but could be one, or a combination of many factors causing the problem. It is a doctor's job to help the patient identify these possible causes to create a treatment plan. It is important to explore all possible causes before jumping to any conclusions.

The most simple, most well accepted cause of acid reflux is the **production of too much acid** in the stomach. As food enters the stomach, it triggers the release of stomach acid into the mix to begin breaking down the food into smaller particles. The amount that is released is usually dependent on how much food, and what type of food needs to be broken down. For example, low fiber foods and simple sugars like refined flour products are easily broken down into their smallest form and therefore do not require much stomach acid to digest. More complex particles, like animal proteins or high fiber foods will need a bit more acid to break them down. If this recognition system gets out of whack, food may trigger a release of stomach acid that is not appropriate for the food. When the food is quickly dissolved by an overwhelming amount of acid, it is released from the stomach into the small intestine. If the stomach is still producing acid on an empty stomach, it is likely to cause a problem. In the case where too much acid is produced, reflux symptoms are more likely to occur.

The pharmaceutical industry thrives on this concept, as there are several prescription and over the counter remedies that work by reducing stomach acid. These options will be discussed in more detail later. The theory is that if there were less stomach acid altogether, there would be less that would enter the esophagus, therefore relieving symptoms and causing less damage.

Functional issues leading to GERD:

There are also many functional problems in the esophagus and stomach region that can lead to acid reflux. When food enters the mouth and slides down the esophagus toward the stomach, the lower esophageal sphincter (LES) opens to let the bolus (chewed mass of food) into the stomach, then close quickly behind the bolus, protecting the esophagus from any acid that tries to enter. The LES is finely tuned to open at the specific moment the bolus reaches it. If there is any confusion in this signaling, if there were nerve damage, for example, the LES may begin to open at inappropriate times, giving stomach acid the opportunity to enter the esophagus.

The lower esophageal sphincter can also become distorted or misshapen, which does not allow it to close completely. This can either be a structural issue, or can be caused by issues with the stomach. When there is increased pressure in the stomach, it pushes up on the lower esophageal sphincter, opening it slightly. When the seal of the sphincter is compromised, any bit of acid that splashes up through it will cause a burning, painful sensation we call heartburn. The pressure can be caused by excess food in the stomach caused by eating too much too fast. There may also be a functional issue with the stomach, which causes it to empty slower, allowing food to build up, causing the pressure.

A hiatal hernia is another possible cause of consistent reflux. A hiatal hernia happens when there is a larger than normal opening in the diaphragm where the esophagus pokes through to meet the stomach. This extra space allows a portion of the stomach to protrude through, causing extra pressure on the lower esophageal sphincter. In this case, there is a higher chance of acid entering the esophagus.

A hiatal hernia can happen at birth, or develop over time, and can range in size, leading to different symptoms. Most hernias are harmless and go unnoticed unless a doctor suspects it is the cause of symptoms. The majority of cases can be managed with diet change, but more severe cases can be fixed with surgery.

Stress and Acid Reflux

Stress seems to be a common culprit in a number of body ailments. It can cause headaches that turn to migraines, create fatigue, muscle aches, high blood pressure and a number of other problems, including acid reflux and GERD. According to a 2011 study reported on healthline.com, there is a strong correlation between work-induced stress and the incidence of GERD. Participants reported a greater incidence of GERD during times of stress. This study was completed in Norway, with over 40,000 people. They also reported that low job satisfaction was a common thread.

Another study in 1993 shows that people who are more anxious reported a higher severity of symptoms than people who were generally relaxed. Interestingly, the same study found no correlation between these increased feelings of discomfort and a tangible increase in stomach acid. This leads to the theory that stress must have some effect on receptors in the cells of tissue that makes them more sensitive to stimuli, creating the illusion of more symptoms. The doctors theorize that stress somehow turns up sensory receptors in the brain, causing more of a reaction than would normally be induced by a small amount of acid in the esophagus. It proves that symptoms can appear to be exaggerated during stressful times.

Note that the patients involved in this study already reported having symptoms of acid reflux, and that this was a study to determine the role of stress and increasing symptoms of GERD. It does not propose that stress causes acid reflux, necessarily, just that symptoms can appear worse if stress is a factor.

Also, these studies are limited in that they have only reviewed the result of acute stress on acid reflux, like exposure to freezing temperatures or loud, annoying noises in controlled environments. They did not test chronic, consistent stress that can be caused by a strained living situation, financial problems, illness, or long-term problems at work. While acute stresses do exist, the majority of people suffer from long term, deep seeded stressors over time.

While none of the previous study found an increase in stomach acid as a result of stress, one interesting study from 1990 found a correlation with stress-induced increases is stomach acid. It found that people with certain personality traits respond differently to stress, and this response either increases or decreases the production of stomach acid. They found that people who are generally laid back, analytically thinking people tend to have decreased stomach acid when exposed to acute stressors. On the contrary, people who are more emotional and quick to react have elevated stomach acid when stress is introduced. This shows again that there is something more going on with stress and acid reflux, yet the causality is still unclear. More testing will need to be done to clarify this link.

To consider another side of the story, we also know that breathing changes as a result of stress. While a calm, resting person will take long, deep breaths, a person under stress will begin to take shallow, short breaths. The response is as old as the human race. In times of acute stress, labeled the "fight or flight" response, early humans would need to increase the oxygen entering the body in order to prepare for a possible "fight or flight" situation. In response to stress of possible harm or death, the heart rate quickens and breathing quickens in order to supply more oxygen to muscles, including the heart. This is an involuntary body function, so there is really no control over it unless you are aware it is occurring, any you consciously try to control your breathing.

The unfortunate side effect of shallow breathing is a decrease in strength in the muscles that surround the lower esophageal sphincter. Deep breathing allows these muscles to stretch to their maximum, and then contract. Shallow breathing uses only a small amount of the muscle capacity to work. It would be like doing a bicep curl at the gym and only flexing the muscle half way. The whole muscle is not being worked out, therefore, it weakens over time.

This is a good theory to help explain why stress leads to acid reflux. When chronic stress is present, the likelihood of shallow breathing increases. The muscles around the lower esophageal sphincter weaken, leaving the lower esophageal sphincter unsupported, and ready to let in unwanted stomach acid.

Bacteria and GERD

Emerging science is beginning to pinpoint the microbiome, a collection of multiple beneficial bacterial strains living in the gut, as a cause of pressure. It is well known that a variety of bacteria call the gastrointestinal system home. They provide a number of services to the body in exchange for space to live. Bacteria aid in the breakdown and absorption of vitamins and minerals, and help regulate the digestive process. Good, non-harmful strains of bacteria in large colonies help to keep smaller colonies of harmful bacteria in check. They act as an extension to the immune system. This is why yogurt is recommended to help digestive issues. The bacteria present in cultured yogurt help increase the colonies of good bacteria living in the gut, therefore aiding in the digestive process and maintaining the populations of harmful bugs.

Bacteria feed on a number of nutrients, but the most popular is simple sugars broken down from carbohydrate rich foods like pasta, bread and fruit. As the bacteria feed on these nutrients, they create gas as a byproduct. The more simple sugars there are to feed on, the more gas the colony will produce. The gases have nowhere to go but up, settling in the stomach, building pressure. When the lower esophageal sphincter opens to relieve some pressure, it lets the opportunistic stomach acid in, reaching and damaging the esophageal lining.

While beneficial bacteria help the body break down food, harmful strains, like Heliobacter pylori (H. Pylori for short) causes more stomach acid to be produced, causing or exacerbating acid reflux symptoms. The human body has a long history of exposure to H. Pylori, and therefore knows how to rid itself of it. H. Pylori are sensitive to stomach acid and thrive in a neutral or alkaline environment. Knowing this, the body increases the release of stomach acid in response to the presence of the bacteria. H. Pylori is a tough bug to get rid of, so the stomach acid is typically elevated for long periods of time, leading to consistent reflux symptoms. As the stomach cells are exposed to more acid than normal for a long period of time, peptic ulcers begin to develop. If left untreated, the ulcers bleed, leaking much-needed blood from the body. If persistent, nutrient deficiencies and other major problems develop through loss of blood. Not to mention the condition is very painful. Shooting, stabbing pain is a common complaint. Along with stomach acid reducing agents, a patient is likely to need antibiotics to help the body rid itself of the H. Pylori infection.

Chapter 3:
Treatments for Occasional Acid Reflux and GERD

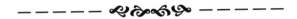

Most people have acid reflux symptoms from time to time, and there are several dietary changes that can be made to avoid the occasional flare up. The most common cause of occasional reflux is over eating, especially eating too much of a certain trigger food. Triggers will vary from person to person, and just because a food seems to cause it once, does not mean it will happen again.

Evidence of acid reflux triggers is varies widely, but some of the most common are as follows:

- Spicy or strong flavored foods like onion and garlic

- Chocolate

- Coffee

- Alcohol

- High acid foods like citrus or tomato, including tomato sauce

- Caffeinated drinks like soda

- High carbohydrate foods

Dietary changes:

If you start suffering more often, it would be a good idea to avoid some of these common triggers to see if symptoms are relieved. Common practice is to completely eliminate possible triggers until no symptoms persist. Foods can then be added back in one at a time until symptoms return.

Avoid Overeating: Overeating is a common cause of reflux. As explained before, overeating can cause pressure on the lower esophageal sphincter, giving the opportunistic gastric juices a chance to splash up onto the esophageal lining. A simple solution is to eat smaller, more frequent meals throughout the day, and avoiding overstuffing yourself. Aim to eat a small meal or snack every 3-4 hours to avoid eating very large meals when you are famished.

Mindful eating is a great tool to use to avoid eating too much. The goal is to allow your body time to digest and signal you when it truly full. With the introduction of super size portions in today's society, this signaling is often ignored. Getting back in touch with the physiology of your own hunger cues will prevent overeating, and can prevent acid reflux. Here are some tips to get started:

- Serve only a small portion of the meal

- Take small, deliberate bites

- Chew fully, about 30 times, before swallowing

- Put your fork down between bites

- Allow your stomach 20 minutes to settle before deciding if you are hungry for seconds

Meal timing also has a huge effect on acid reflux symptoms. Many acid reflux sufferers notice that their symptoms mainly occur, or are more severe, at night. This is for good reason. If the esophageal sphincter is slightly open for any reason, laying down to go to sleep causes a problem. Gravity will naturally bring more stomach acid to the top of the stomach, making it ready to enter the esophagus should the sphincter open. If the sphincter remains open, symptoms will persist as long as you are laying down. Try not to eat for a few hours before bed, giving your stomach time to flush out any unused acid.

If acid reflux does occur mainly at night, many find relief by propping their head up with an extra pillow to reduce the effects of gravity. However, many complain of a stiff neck or inability to sleep due to their body position. In case of persistent night time reflux and neck pain, some report propping up the head of their bed to create a downward slope, defying gravity.

If changing portion size and meal timing doesn't seem to help, changing the types of foods eaten can help. When the underlying cause of your reflux is driven by gut bacteria, changing the proportion of foods you eat is very important. Think about a standard meal of meat, starch and vegetable (let's say steak, potato and broccoli). Most people choose to treat themselves to a large steak, a large baked potato loaded with butter, sour cream or cheese, and a small serving of broccoli, just for color. A large baked potato actually contains several servings of carbohydrate more than is appropriate for most people. Quickly giving your body, and your bacteria a large load of carbohydrates will create a large amount of gas very quickly, which, as explained above, will push on the lower esophageal sphincter and cause acid reflux.

Changing the proportion of the meal to be mostly protein from the steak, a lower carb veggie like broccoli, and less potato, drastically reduces the amount of fuel available to the bacterial colony, therefore decreasing gas build up and reflux symptoms. Cutting your carbohydrate intake in half can quickly reduce symptoms. If the difference is not apparent, eliminating high carb foods like potato, pasta and bread for a short experimental period may be necessary. Consult with a knowledgeable dietitian or nutritionist to help determine what your nutrient needs are and to develop a plan for dealing with your acid reflux. See a sample 3-day meal plan later on.

Chapter 4:
Over the counter and natural remedies

————— ✤✤✤✤ —————

There will be occasions where overeating occurs, and acid reflux symptoms flare up, especially if you are experimenting with trigger foods. For immediate relief, there are several options, ranging from over the counter acid neutralizers to home remedies people swear by. Let's start with options found at the drugstore:

OTC remedies

- Acid neutralizers- products like Tums or Maalox contain alkaline chemicals that neutralize stomach acid immediately. These are the best products for relief once your symptoms have already started. As the pH rises, it causes less damage to esophageal cells, reducing the pain and burning sensation. The main ingredient in Tums is calcium carbonate, while the active ingredients in Maalox are aluminum hydroxide, magnesium hydroxide and simethicone. Its thick milky consistency coats the lining of the esophagus, protecting it from unruly gastric juices. Maalox is a multi-purpose product meant to reduce upset stomach and gas as well. Pick the product that will help your symptoms with the least amount of unnecessary ingredients.

- Acid reducers- products like Prilosec or Tagamet utilize chemicals to shut down the production of acid. While these products are effective, they do not work immediately, and can take up to two weeks to relieve symptoms. Their purpose is to provide relief while the underlying cause of the reflux is diagnosed. These products are not meant to be used long term. Once these options are stopped, symptoms are likely to return if the source of the problem has not been determined.

Natural alternatives to medication

- Baking soda-a natural source of sodium bicarbonate, the active ingredient in Tums, baking soda can be a quick, cost effective remedy for occasional acid reflux. A teaspoon mixed with a glass of water swiftly neutralizes acid and relieves symptoms. While it may not taste great, like the flavored over the counter Tums brand, it will provide similar relief. If you really can't get past the taste, try adding a splash of juice to sweeten the mixture.

- Dairy products-much like Maalox, dairy products like milk, cream or yogurt are thick, viscous substances that are able to coat the lining of the esophagus, protecting it from acid.

- Gum- studies show that increasing saliva can help dilute acid built up in the lower esophagus. Chewing gum stimulates the salivary glands in the mouth to produce excess saliva, which, when swallowed, helps wash some of the stomach acid out, decreasing symptoms.

- Bitters- a group of bitter herbs that are said to stimulate gastric juice production can help restore balance in your microbiota. Herbs include ginger, hops and peppermint. A word of warning: Bitters are usually associated as a trigger for acid reflux symptoms. This is not appropriate for immediate relief of existing symptoms, but may help if eaten before a meal to stimulate acid production before food enters the gut.

Chapter 5:
Activities for symptom relief

————— ❧❦❧ —————

Taking a pill or other home remedy is a great quick fix, but there are other alternative tricks to help prevent and relieve symptoms to try.

Deep breathing exercises

Who knew that something as simple as deep breathing could help relieve symptoms of acid reflux? A 2011 study from *The American Journal of Gastroenterology reports that specific breathing exercises targeting the diaphragm, the muscles surrounding the esophageal sphincter, strengthening it over time, reducing problematic acid reflux symptoms. By relearning to breathe, pressure on the sphincter decreases, eliminating symptoms.*

There is no magic set of directions to start deep breathing exercise. Begin by sitting or laying in a comfortable position. Breathe normally for a few minutes, and recognize where you feel your breath. Place one hand on your chest and one hand on your belly. Does the air fill into your chest or your belly? Next, begin the deep breathing exercise. Simply start by sitting up straight, and breathing from your belly and not your chest. If your hand is on your belly and stomach, your chest should not move, and air should enter your belly as you breathe in rather than your chest. Breathe in fully, until no more air can enter your lungs. Then, breathe out slowly and completely, until you feel strained expelling air.

Activities for symptom relief

This straining helps strengthen the diaphragm, supporting the esophageal sphincter. The 2011 study in The American Journal of Gastroenterology reports that most participants experienced at least some symptom relief, better quality of life after nine months. Major improvements were made in symptoms occurring when patients were laying down to sleep at night, and reflux related to sleep apnea through the night.

Participants practiced conscious deep breathing techniques for 30 minutes per day over nine months. The 30 minutes does not have to be all at once. It can be done in five or ten minute increments throughout the day. It can be done sitting, standing or lying down. All it takes is a few minutes of concentration. Breathing is an involuntary function, something we do without thinking. In order to alter the way you breathe, it takes conscious effort.

Excessive deep breathing can cause you to become light headed and dizzy, so if these symptoms start while doing the exercise, stop the session and begin breathing normally. You may begin again once symptoms subside. Several sources report success with compliance, and remembering to complete the exercises, when they are done first thing in the morning, even before getting out of bed. Try practicing deep breathing as part of your wake up ritual. You will exercise your diaphragm and get a boost in energy from the increased oxygen intake first thing in the morning.

While symptom relief may not be immediate or complete, the best part about this remedy is that it costs nothing, and has no negative side effects. The scientific evidence behind this method is lacking, but muscle imagery shows that as muscles relax and the body calms, the esophageal sphincter responds and contracts. Deep breathing has also been shown to reduce *stress, another possible cause of your reflux symptoms. Why not add it to your daily regimen to see if it makes a difference in both your heartburn symptoms and your stress levels?*

Drink plenty of water: Drinking water can help dilute and neutralize stomach acid and wash excess acid that has entered the esophagus back down into the stomach. This process reduces the immediate symptoms, and decreases the damage done by acid that remains stagnant in the esophagus. Several sources report that increasing water intake throughout the day can help relieve symptoms.

It appears, however, that timing of drinking water is everything. The ideal time to drink extra water is right before a meal. Waiting to have water after or during a meal fills the stomach, and delays gastric emptying, causing food to build up. This creates pressure on the esophageal sphincter, preventing it from fully closing. Drinking excess water with meals also dilutes the acid at a time where it is needed in full strength to aid in digestion and sterilization of food particles before they enter the blood stream. You must let the acid do the job it was intended to do. Undigested food particles can cause stomach and lower gastrointestinal upset as the concentrated molecules attract water into the GI system to dilute it. This can cause almost immediate symptoms of gastric flushing, diarrhea, gas and bloating. These symptoms can be urgent and unpleasant. Letting the stomach acid do its job can prevent this from happening and keeps the system moving as it was meant to. Have a glass before your meal, then about a half hour after, a little bit more to wash down any remaining acid from the esophagus.

Most resources recommend at least eight full glasses of water per day. Depending on your average water intake to begin with, this may be a lofty goal. If eight glasses seems excessive, try by increasing by a glass or two a day and build up to eight glasses per day. You certainly don't want to be in and out of the bathroom every half hour, so find a good balance. Be sure to monitor acid reflux symptoms as you decrease your intake to determine if it is making a difference.

Besides acid reflux, increasing water keeps the GI system in top shape, increasing regularity and eliminating symptoms of constipation. Water is consider the 'universal solvent' and is good for every cell in your body. If your acid reflux symptoms don't seem to subside by drinking more water, you will likely see differences in other areas of your body as well, so keep it up!

Some people struggle drinking water by itself. While plain water can get boring, it really is the best option. Flavors, like lemon or lime juice can be added to make it more appealing. Avoid adding excess sugars from powdered lemonade or iced tea mixes as the additional sugar can cause gas to be produced by gut bacteria. Carbonated beverages like soda or seltzer water should be skipped if they are acid reflux triggers. Coffee provides water as well, but caffeine can be a reflux trigger, and since it acts as a diuretic, actually pulls more water out of the body. Decaffeinated teas could be a good option if you need to avoid caffeine, but would still like a flavor kick. Licorice tea is a good choice because it increases the mucus production in the esophagus. As it builds up, it coats the cell lining, giving a layer of protection against unruly stomach acid.

Adding a splash of lemon or lime seems counterintuitive, as it is acidic, but that could actually work in your favor. Presence of acid in the stomach actually shuts down the proton pumps that excrete acid because it senses the pH is as low as it should be. However, use acidic juices in moderation because if ulcers exist in the stomach, or damage in the esophagus is extensive, the excess acid will irritate an already irritated cell lining.

Another water option, believe it or not, is alkaline water. Certain brands of bottled water report their products have an alkaline pH, which can help balance out stomach acid. While most evidence is anecdotal, it does make sense that an alkaline substance will help balance out an acid. Whether it relieves symptoms completely, and for how long is unknown.

Apple cider vinegar

Touted as the cure-all for all that ails you, apple cider vinegar can be a great home remedy for acid reflux. Apple cider vinegar helps neutralize acid in the stomach. On its own, apple cider vinegar is very strong, just like distilled white vinegar. It should not be taken alone, as the concentrated dose can actually damage the esophageal lining, exactly the opposite effect we're looking for. Instead, dilute about a tablespoon of apple cider vinegar in an 8oz glass of water. A good daily regimen to try is a morning glass of water with apple cider vinegar. This can set your stomach off on the right foot, in a more alkaline state. Lots of people claim to find immediate relief of symptoms by trying this remedy at onset of acid reflux.

Besides acid reflux relief, apple cider vinegar is thought to aid in digestion further along in the system. The potassium in the vinegar helps lower blood pressure, in turn leading to lower risk of heart disease. Taking apple cider vinegar at meal time has been shown to curb hunger and increase feelings of satiety. This can lead to better blood sugar control, reducing the risk of diabetes, and aiding in weight loss over time. With all of these possible positive benefits, why not try apple cider vinegar in your daily routine to increase overall health.

Increasing physical activity

The recommendation for exercise is a double edged sword. Vigorous exercise like running and jumping can stir up stomach acid, causing it to splash against the esophageal sphincter, and enter the esophagus should the sphincter be open. Vigorous exercise is not recommended after a meal, for a number of reasons, but specifically because this would be the time that the most stomach acid will be present in the body. Swearing off all exercise because of acid reflux symptoms puts you at risk for disease related to sedentary lifestyle, like obesity, diabetes, and heart disease. It is necessary to exercise to keep your whole body healthy and keep weight in control.

The general recommendation is to do exercises that are only mildly vigorous and that can be done in an upright position. For example, walking or speed walking will be better than running or sprinting. Weight training exercises done in an upright position, like squats and arm curls are better than push ups or sit ups, in which you will be in a horizontal position. Low impact cardio, like using an elliptical, may be a good starting point. Try not to eat within a couple hours of exercise to avoid peak acid production times.

Many studies show that even a small decrease in weight can help improve acid reflux symptoms, and exercise in general helps as well. Low impact practices like yoga or Tai Chi are good exercises to try, as they incorporate traditional cardio exercise, weight bearing exercises, balance and flexibility training and conscious deep breathing techniques. However, avoid floor exercises should they may trigger symptoms.

Exercise after your last meal can help settle the stomach and decrease likelihood of symptoms. Studies show that people who have their last meal about three hours before bedtime and participate in light exercise, like a walk around the neighborhood after dinner, tend to have the lowest incidence of acid reflux at bedtime. Participants in this study also report sleeping better, likely due to decreased symptoms during the night.

Exercise has been proven to lower stress levels in the body as well. Several studies have proven that increased stress can increase the body's sensitivity to the pain and discomfort that acid reflux causes. Getting some regular exercise, and even more when stress is high at work or at home can help relieve symptoms of GERD. While exercise takes care of the psychosomatic symptoms of GERD, providing some relief, it is still important to find the root cause of your reflux. Just because you don't feel the symptoms as strongly does not mean the acid is not damaging the lining of your esophagus.

Chapter 6:
Prescription remedies for
long term symptoms

$----- \, \mathscr{eeeee} \, -----$

When acid reflux occurs consistently for a long period of time despite dietary changes and other home remedies, it is time to speak with your doctor. They can run the necessary tests to determine what the underlying cause of your symptoms are. You can decide together whether a prescription medication is a good solution. Here are the options:

Proton pump inhibitors: This class of medication is the most common. It includes pantoprazole (Protonix), lansoprazole (Prevacid), esomeprazole (Nexium) and omeprazole (Prilosec). These medicines work by shutting down proton pumps in stomach lining cells, decreasing the amount of acid being produced by the stomach. It actually emits acid signals in the stomach, which trick the proton pumps into thinking there is enough acid in the stomach, which then deactivates them. While it may not get after the root cause of your problem, it can be used to give the esophagus and stomach time to heal without excess acid continually irritating the inflamed areas. Several proton pump inhibitors have been approved for over the counter use in the past few years. It is now possible to try Prevacid and Prilosec without a prescription, however, use should be instructed by your doctor.

H2 blockers: These medications also work to suppress acid production, but they do so by attaching to histamine receptors in stomach lining cells. Histamine signals proton pumps to create more acid, so when H2 blockers keep these receptors busy, histamine does not have the opportunity to relay this message to them. Acid production will then slow, temporarily reducing symptoms. There are several variations of H2 blockers, including cimetidine (Tagamet), ranitidine (Zantac), famotidine (Pepcid) and nizatidine (Axid). Some of these medications are available over the counter as well. Commonly known brands like Pepcid and Tagamet have been approved for use without a prescription. As with any new treatment, consult your doctor before beginning treatment.

Both proton pump inhibitors and H2 blockers are good options to help reduce symptoms short term. There are options available over the counter, but most insurance companies cover these classes of medications with a prescription. Over the counter options range in price, generally between ten and thirty dollars per pack. Insurance could save you money on a large supply for little to no cost out of pocket.

Chapter 7:
Side effects of prescription medications
— — — — — ✧❦✧❦✧ — — — —

Minor side effects of PPIs include headache, and a range of gastrointestinal issues such as diarrhea, nausea, gas, abdominal pain, constipation, dry mouth and drowsiness according to Nexium's website. To be clear, other versions of PPI medications have similar side effects, this is not a specific problem with Nexium alone. Only one to three percent of patients decide to stop taking the medication, according to Consumer Reports' 2013 review of acid reflux medications. It is not surprising that these gastrointestinal side effects are present. If stomach acid is not present to help break down food particles as it should, partially processed food gets pushed into the small intestine, which is used to food being delivered in a broken down, readily absorbable form. The small intestine will struggle to absorb food, and large particles will pass through the system as is, creating unwanted symptoms of discomfort, pain and bloating.

According to Nexium's website, their product, esomeprazole has a long list of long term problems associated with it. Let's go through each issue:

Increased risk of infection

The most obvious long term problem would be susceptibility to infection. Because the primary function of stomach acid is to act as first line defender for the immune system, decreasing its action puts the body at greater risk for infection. As discussed earlier, opportunistic bacteria like H. Pylori can take hold if there is not enough acid to deter its colonization.

According to a study published by ...in 2011, low stomach acid is correlated with the colonization of Salmonella, Campylobacter jejuni, Escherichia coli, Clostridium difficile, Vibrio cholerae and Listeria, all of which are foodborne illnesses that cause gastrointestinal symptoms ranging from upset stomach to coma and death.

These bacterial strains are able to get past stomach acid and cause infection in healthy people with average amounts of stomach acid. As stomach acid is reduced, the chance of infection increases, and the longer this first line immune defense is suppressed, the higher the likelihood of developing an issue.

People with low acid, either by natural causes, or through the use of acid suppressing medications should be extra cautious in preparing their foods in a safe manner. Make sure to cook foods thoroughly, for the correct amount of time to kill bacteria. Avoid eating raw foods as much as possible, including salad greens like lettuce, that can easily be contaminated with Listeria, a water borne bacteria that is common on vegetables.

Decrease in vitamin absorption:

It is well-documented that stomach acid begins the digestive process, and aids the absorption of several essential vitamins and minerals. The most affected nutrients are Vitamin B12 and magnesium. Vitamin B12 requires intrinsic factor, a component of gastric juices in order to be absorbed into the bloodstream. It must bind to intrinsic factor before a cell will let it enter. Vitamin B12 has many functions in the body, including regulation of the nervous system, energy production, and it is a building block to creating DNA and RNA, the genetic material necessary to make new cells, most specifically red blood cells that deliver oxygen to tissue in the body. If B12 is not absorbed, neurological issues can develop. The most common symptom is fatigue, related to the slowed process of energy production and the decreased oxygen delivery by red blood cells. Symptoms of nerve damage range from tingling in the extremities to loss of feeling. Most cases of B12 deficiency can be caught before serious problems occur. Deficiencies can be corrected by supplementing orally, but in the case of low stomach acid, oral supplement will go unabsorbed if they have no intrinsic factor to guide them into cells. Injections of B12 are also available to bypass the GI tract and deliver it straight to the bloodstream.

Magnesium absorption is commonly low without stomach acid as well. Magnesium is a necessary mineral, responsible for hundreds of enzymatic reactions in the body. Enzymes are the 'keys' to chemical reactions that get things done in the body. Think of enzymes as the car that drives you to work. Without it, you will not get where you need to go. Enzymes, like cars, require fuel to get them working. While there are several cofactors (the fuel), magnesium is one of the most commonly used by enzymes in the muscle and nervous systems. Magnesium is also important in blood pressure and blood glucose regulation. Low magnesium levels can lead to diabetes, heart disease and a plethora of neurological disorders. Low magnesium may also have an effect on kidney function, as will be explained a little later.

With the influx of new prescription drugs flooding the shelves, you've likely seen commercials advertising miracle drugs that eliminate symptoms of acid reflux when taken regularly. While this is true, it's important to realize that the motivation of these companies is to sell their product. They do not make diagnoses, nor have the ability to monitor every patient their medications go out to. They prompt medical professionals to try their products with patients who can't find relief. It is up to the doctor to decide what, if any, long term medications are appropriate. It's also up to the doctor to limit the amount of time a patient is on medication to avoid any unnecessary complications.

Without singling out any specific medication in particular, long term acid reducers actually have short-sighted goals in mind. Yes, these products will reduce the overall acid your stomach produces and relieve symptoms. But, as we talked about earlier, your stomach produces acid for a reason, and if it is overproducing gastric juices, there is likely a good reason behind it. Taking medications that reduce acid only mask the underlying cause of the overproduction in the first place.

Without further investigation, a patient who begins an acid reflux medication will likely need to stay on it for the rest of their life to avoid the return of symptoms.

Bone density issues, Bone fractures: If you were to search possible side effects of PPI medications, you would find claims showing decreased bone density and increased risk of bone fracture in patients who have been on this method of therapy long term. Stomach acid helps facilitate the absorption of several vitamins and minerals, including calcium. When stomach acid is suppressed, the absorption of calcium decreases, leaving little available for bones to grow or make repairs. While most calcium is stored in bone, it actually has several uses outside the human skeleton. Calcium helps send nerve signals to muscles, including the heart. While bones are important, if there is a lack of calcium in the blood, it will be removed from bone to use to keep the heart functioning properly. The goal is to get enough calcium in the diet to support the heart and other functions and not pull calcium from the bones. Suppressing stomach acid can greatly reduce the amount of calcium absorbed. This is especially troublesome for someone who is already lacking this mineral in their diet.

While several studies have shown a positive correlation with long term PPI use and bone density issues, and more specifically, incidence of hip fractures, other studies show little to no correlation. According to a review done by the Federal Drug Administration (FDA), no evidence exists that the risk of bone fracture increases with PPI use in normally healthy individuals. However, there are correlations with PPI use and bone fracture in individuals who are at greater risk for low bone density and bone fracture due to other factors. It is unclear whether the progression of bone loss or likelihood of bone fracture increases with PPI use in someone who is already susceptible to these issues. So unfortunately, the results of these studies don't tell us much.

While H2 blocking medications essentially have the same effect as PPIs, the reduction of overall stomach acid, you would think that they would also carry warnings about the risk of osteoporosis or bone fracture. At this point, the FDA has not been able to find the same correlation with H2 blockers and bone loss, even though absorption of calcium does decrease as the pH of the stomach increases and becomes more alkaline. Most likely, we will hear similar claims regarding H2 blockers in the next few years.

The increased likelihood of osteoporosis with long term medication use is concerning, but there are ways to make sure you are at least getting enough calcium from the diet to make up for less being absorbed. Supplementation of calcium in tablet or capsule form is probably the easiest way to increase free calcium in the body. Also, including more rich sources of calcium from the diet helps as well. Dark, leafy greens like kale and spinach are good sources of calcium, as well as from milk, yogurt, cheese, and other dairy products.

A word of caution, however. Increasing dairy products in the diet can lead to constipation and stomach upset in large amounts. If you are not used to eating a lot of dairy, slowly increase and note any adverse symptoms. If you experience GI upset, supplementing your calcium will be the best solution.

Kidney problems (acute interstitial nephritis): The human kidney is largely responsible for filtering the blood, ridding it of toxins and excess vitamins and minerals. Once through the kidney, any substance that needs to leave the body does so through the urinary tract system. The end result is the excretion of urine. The color of urine is dependent on what substances are being excreted by the kidneys. Urinalysis tests are used to monitor presence of toxins or drugs that have entered the body, and can also monitor the overall function of the kidneys.

Several studies have linked PPI use with acute kidney failure, especially in those whose kidneys are already compromised. Scientists have pinpointed the decrease in Magnesium absorption as the probable cause behind kidney dysfunction. Just like with calcium, stomach acid helps aid in the absorption of Magnesium as well. As stomach acid declines, so does the absorption of Magnesium.

There is conflicting information regarding possible treatments of kidney disease when it comes to magnesium. On one hand, any additional vitamins or minerals that are taken in need to be processed through the kidney, causing increased stress on the organ. However, the relationship between magnesium and calcium in the kidney also needs to be considered. Magnesium and calcium both compete for the same receptors in the kidney. If there is a shortage of magnesium, the kidney will process more calcium if it is in good supply. Excess calcium buildup can cause problems like kidney stones or gall stones, a condition in which calcium crystallizes in large pieces. When these pieces come loose, they need to pass through the urinary tract system. These large particles scratch the lining of the system on their way through, causing pain and bleeding. If severe enough, it can lead to infection.

A buildup of magnesium, on the other hand, does not happen, as excess magnesium is simply flushed out of the system. The goal of kidney treatment is to counteract the deposit of calcium using adequate amounts of magnesium. What is unclear though, is the correlation between PPI use and kidney failure. Low stomach acid inhibits the absorption of both calcium and magnesium.

Again, like with claims of bone density loss, PPI medications are singled out and H2 blockers have not been found to share the same side effects.

Certain types of lupus erythematosus

The FDA does not recognize lupus as directly caused by PPI medications, but it is listed as a possible side effect on several PPI med lists. Lupus is an auto immune disease, meaning that the immune system attacks parts of the body because it falsely recognizes certain normal cells as foreign. Auto immune diseases take many forms, including thyroid disorders, arthritis and skin conditions like psoriasis and eczema.

There are many symptoms of lupus, including decreases in energy, headaches, joint pain and circulation issues, such as Reynaud's syndrome, in which the tips of the fingers tingle and turn white or blue from lack of circulation. All of these symptoms are congruent with several other conditions, and could be due to a number of other underlying issues.

Classic symptoms that set Lupus apart are rashes across the face, usually on the cheeks and nose, resembling a butterfly. These rashes can also appear on the back. Diagnosis can be difficult because problems will occur at the site in the body that the immune system is attacking.

There are connections with autoimmune diseases like lupus with food allergies, specifically, pro-inflammatory foods like gluten, dairy and soy, although any food could pose a problem. This would be specific to an individual. As an offending food passes through the GI system, it causes damage to the cells lining stomach and small intestine. Certain foods stimulate the release of zonulin, originally discovered by Dr. Alessio Fassano, which causes the pathways existing between cells to open, allowing compounds into cells. These pathways usually only open up when essential nutrients are present, so they may enter the bloodstream.

The release of zonulin on a constant basis, let's say, if an offending food is consumed on a regular basis, the pathways always stay open, which gives the opportunity for substances that would normally not be allowed into the bloodstream in. The immune system then reacts, sensing a foreign substance. When the immune system is heightened for long periods of time, it begins to start attacking cells in the body, leading to degradation of the organ cells it is attacking.

Because symptoms typically don't develop overnight, it can be difficult to diagnose an autoimmune disorder as the problem.

PPIs are typically associated with joint pain and the skin symptoms, like rashes and blisters. The exact mechanism that leads PPIs to this syndrome are unknown at this point. Most patients with this side effect find relief from symptoms when they stop taking the medication. Instances of this side effect are rare. If symptoms similar to lupus start to develop after onset of medication, make sure to speak to your doctor to diagnose the cause.

Too little stomach acid

It may seem counterintuitive, but emerging science is making a case that too little stomach acid can actually be responsible for acid reflux. There are two working theories that compound this issue. First, the esophageal sphincter is programmed to close when it detects acid. This is the natural response to close to protect the esophagus while the stomach works on digesting food. When too little stomach acid is produced in response to food, the esophagus is not prompted to close all of the way, leading to symptoms.

If this is the case, then long-term acid inhibiting medications may actually be compounding the problem at hand. Second, stomach acid is present to help kill of any harmful bacteria, and, in some cases, beneficial bacteria that has been allowed to thrive and has overstayed its welcome. If there is not enough stomach acid to keep bacterial levels in check, colonies thrive, producing more gas byproduct as they eat and multiply.

As the gas builds, the acid reflux worsens, and there is no increase in stomach acid to balance the bacteria back out.

While beneficial bacteria causes little threat to health besides the acid reflux, opportunistic bacteria like H. Pylori, Salmonella or Shigella that thrives in a low acid environment will be allowed to colonize and cause systemic illness. Lowering the body's natural immune protection opens up many opportunities for sneaky bacteria and viruses to take hold, leading to a decline in health over time.

One of the leading experts in this method of treatment is Chris Kresser, M.S., L.Ac. He explains that it can take a long time to balance your gut microbiota to restore calm and reduce symptoms of reflux, but it is possible with the "three Rs":

1. **Reduce** factors that promote bacterial overgrowth and low stomach acid.

2. **Replace** stomach acid, enzymes and nutrients that aid digestion and are necessary for health.

3. **Restore** beneficial bacteria and a healthy mucosal lining in the gut.

The use of synthesized digestive enzyme supplements can help mimic missing stomach acid to aid digestion and begin to get bacterial overgrowth in check. This in tandem with reducing the food source for harmful bacteria (mainly carbohydrates and sugars) reduces overall populations. It is also helpful to supplement with probiotics to take the place of less beneficial bacteria that may have populated the gut before. There is only so much space in the gut, so flooding it with new colonies of beneficial bacteria will help ensure that less desirable, even harmful strains will not have space to recolonize.

Kresser adds that certain types of sugars cause exacerbated symptoms. The type of sugar sensitivity depends on what strains of bacteria are present in the gut, and what types of sugar molecules they thrive on. A low Fermentable Oligosaccharides, Disaccharides, Monosaccharides And Polyols (FODMAP for short) diet is an elimination plan that removes several types of sugars from the diet to reduce symptoms. Foods containing said sugars will be added back in one group at a time to determine which form of sugar seems to trigger the most symptoms. Once pinpointed, the food can be consumed modestly, or not at all to control symptoms.

Costs of medication

Like any over the counter or prescription drug, there are costs to consider when beginning a medication. Is this something you can afford to take on a monthly basis? The good news is, these products have been around long enough that the patents from their original brand-name developers has expired, and generic versions are available from several companies. When there are more choices, the cost of medication drops so companies can stay competitive in the market.

Those price drops become a direct savings to the consumer. Still, there are new versions of medications being developed all the time, and newer is better, at least from a marketing standpoint. Drug company sales reps do a great job convincing doctors that their newest product is the best, and many doctors will try a patient on a newer medication that does not have a generic.

If your doctor writes you a prescription, opt to try a medication that has been on the market longer, and has a generic available. You can save money, and sleep well at night knowing that the longer a medication is on the market, the more opportunity it has to be tested for previously undiscovered side effects. This tried and true product may be safer than the newest option.

Chapter 8:
Diet for acid reflux and GERD

— — — — — ❧❦❧❦ — — — —

This is the part where we take all of the many recommendations discussed in this book and turn them into a usable diet plan. While this plan will be basic so that it will fit the needs of a large group of people, it should be used as a guideline to base your diet plan off of. You will need to consider personal calorie needs. Your current weight, body composition, and activity level should all be included when deciding what an appropriate number of calories is for you.

Personal food allergies and sensitivities should also be monitored. It's very simple. If a specific food is recommended in the following plan that you are allergic to, or have had an adverse reaction to in the past, do not include it in your personal plan. If, after reading the plan are unsure what to do, consult with a registered dietitian or other qualified health professional that can help with tailoring a plan specific to you.

There are several diets, ranging from extreme elimination diets to more manageable plans that shift your dietary habits to a more acid reflux friendly version. It is up to you which plan to try first. If you participate in a cleanse, make sure not to continue longer than recommended, as negative side effects may occur.

The Basics

Avoid foods that can be possible triggers, as well as ones that you know trigger your acid reflux specifically. That common trigger list is as follows:

- Spicy or strong flavored foods like onion and garlic

- Chocolate

- Coffee

- Alcohol

- High acid foods like citrus or tomato

- Caffeinated drinks like soda

- High carbohydrate foods

Detox diet for acid reflux

This plan is meant to be a quick way to relieve symptoms, to cleanse your digestive system and ready it for a new eating plan. There are several variations, but here are a few examples.

- **Apples and apple juice diet**- a two day cleanse, this diet consists of only fresh, organic apples and apple juices. It is easy to find organic apples, but be careful to choose an apple juice that is free of added sugars, artificial sweeteners or preservatives. After two days, transition to fresh, organic fruits and vegetables and brown rice. After 4 days, begin to transition to a normal, reflux friendly diet.

Diet for acid reflux and GERD

- **Vegetable juice cleanse**-this program uses fruits and vegetables that are soothing to the body as a sort of medicine. Making smoothies out of very alkaline vegetables like kale or cabbage can help balance out stomach acid. Truthfully, just about any vegetable will do, aside from high acid varieties like tomatoes. Avoid peppers as well if they are a trigger for you. While there is no time recommendation for this cleanse, drinking a variety of vegetable juices throughout the day, and making sure to include even more veggies at meals can help reduce acid in the stomach. This can be used in combination with the following carb elimination option as well.

- **Carbohydrate elimination**-this elimination is all about figuring out what an appropriate carbohydrate level is for your body. While carbohydrates are a necessary component to a healthy diet, the idea of eliminating the for the sake of reducing acid reflux symptoms is appealing. Should your reflux stem from issues with gas buildup from overeating, or from an unruly colony of gas-producing bacteria, eliminating carbs could be a good option. Simply build your meals around lean meats like beef, chicken and fish. Add a hefty portion of non-starchy vegetables, like salad greens, broccoli, spinach, pretty much anything green. Stay away from grains like bread and pasta, refined sugars found in cookies or ice cream, and starchy vegetables like potatoes and corn. Try this for up to two weeks to get an out of control bacterial colony under control, and the gas production minimized. Begin adding carbohydrates back in slowly after that. Try simple sugars from fruits first. Add items back until you start feeling symptoms starting to return. Back off the carbs until you return to a carbohydrate level your body is comfortable with.

This diet cleanse should be completed for no more than two days, and if you decide to participate, be careful to monitor any symptoms like dizziness, feeling lightheaded, feeling weak, or anything else that is out of the ordinary for you. If present, stop the cleanse immediately and contact your doctor if symptoms persist after transitioning back to a normal diet.

People with diabetes should be especially careful of cleanse and fasting diets because it can cause their blood sugars to drop or spike out of normal ranges. The apple cleanse diet can be especially problematic because you will be taking in a large amount of carbohydrates from the apples and apple juice, and no proteins or fat to help balance it out. Blood sugar numbers are very likely to spike, causing dangerous side effects.

Chapter 9:
3-Day Meal Plan

— — — — — ❧❦❧ — — — —

If diet cleanses or fasting are not for you, creating a more balanced, standard eating pattern can do the trick as well. The following diet example can also be used as a follow up to any of the cleanses described above, or you could simply start here. This plan is simple to follow and does not include any difficult to find ingredients or complicated recipes. The only requirement is that you try your best to adhere to the diet before passing any judgment as to whether it works or not.

This diet combines solutions to all of the possible causes of acid reflux, therefore should be beneficial to you no matter what the situation. The diet is also approved for several other conditions, including heart disease, diabetes, and it may even help you lose a little weight.

Here is your 3-day meal plan to get you started. Keep in mind this plan is based on about a 2000 calorie diet, so adjustments to portion sizes are likely appropriate. Also note that timing of meals is important. Each meal and snack should be no more than 4 hours apart.

Day One:

Breakfast: Two eggs, one slice of whole wheat toast, 1 teaspoon of butter, margarine or oil of choice.

Snack: Small apple, 1 tablespoon of peanut butter.

Lunch: Large salad including mixed greens, cucumbers, carrots (avoid tomato and pepper if triggers), a palm-size piece of grilled chicken, and 1 tablespoon of dressing, (half and half oil and apple cider vinegar).

Snack: Fruit and nut bar of choice, avoiding any fruit triggers if they exist

Dinner: Grilled salmon with sautéed asparagus and no more than half cup brown rice.

Dessert: One half cup mashed banana plus 1 tablespoon peanut butter. Freeze banana then mash for ice cream consistency.

Day Two:

Breakfast: Two to three egg omelet made with steamed broccoli and mushroom. Serve with no more than one half cup of mixed fruit.

Snack: 3 cups of plain, unsalted, unbuttered popcorn plus 1 tablespoon unsalted almonds

Lunch: Lettuce wrap filled with your choice of grilled chicken, fish or steak tips. Add other vegetables of choice. Mayonnaise or oil and apple cider vinegar are great for condiments. Serve with a small serving of fruit.

Snack: 2 tablespoons raisins (or kid size box) plus 1 tablespoon unsalted cashews.

Dinner: Meatloaf served with zucchini noodles coated with a light layer of olive oil. Spice to taste, avoiding reflux triggers.

Dessert: Apple slices from one small apple plus one tablespoon Nutella

Day Three:

Breakfast: No more than one half cup cooked oatmeal (one quarter cup dry) plus 2-3 tablespoons of peanut butter or other nut butter for protein. Add vanilla and cinnamon to taste.

Snack: No more than one half cup melon plus 1 tablespoon unsalted peanuts.

Lunch: Ground beef sautéed with mushrooms, served with no more than one half cup brown rice and side salad.

Snack: Lunchmeat rollups-two slices of lunchmeat of choice, plus one half cup assorted fruit.

Dinner: Roasted chicken (rotisserie) plus a heaping portion of broccoli plus no more than ½ cup mashed potatoes.

Dessert: One half cup frozen mixed berries with 1 tablespoon Nutella.

This plan can easily be carried on long term. Simply use the following ratio guidelines to plan your weekly meals. Use these guidelines to fix your plate.

- One half of the plate should be vegetables, at least for lunch and dinner (it is not always possible to fit them in at breakfast). The best bet is to buy organic vegetables, those which have been grown without the use of artificial insecticides and fertilizers. These products create a host of other issues that have links to cancer and other conditions in the body. Vegetables that come directly from the Earth without anything added are the best.

- One quarter of the plate should be lean protein from chicken, eggs, fish, pork or beef. The best sources of meat are free range or cage free chicken, wild caught fish and grass fed, grass finished beef or pork. The quality of the meat highly depends on what the animals are fed and how they are treated. A diet high in grains will give meat that is high in inflammatory Omega 6 fatty acids and low in anti inflammatory Omega 3 fatty acids. Animals fed their natural source of food, like grass for cows, will have higher Omega 3 content, which is better for the animal and you.

- One quarter (maximum) of the plate should be carbohydrates. Avoid refined and processed grains like bread, pasta and cereals. If you do eat these, whole grain varieties provide more fiber and have a lower glycemic index, meaning they will not have such an effect on your blood sugar. The majority of carbohydrates should come from complex plant sources like starchy vegetables and fruits. However, avoid potatoes and corn, as these have higher concentrations of carbohydrates.

Conclusion

— — — — — ❧❦❧ — — — —

Thank for making it through to the end of this book, let's hope it was informative and able to provide you with all of the tools you need to achieve your goals whatever they may be.

The next step is to make informed decisions regarding the treatment of your acid reflux. Whether your symptoms are new, occasional, consistent or long-lasting, there are options for treatment. While medications and medical procedures are an option, starting by trying simple, inexpensive remedies at home.

Creating lasting diet and lifestyle changes may be all you need to lead a happy, healthy life without the burden of taking medications on a daily basis, and dealing with a number of adverse side effects. Remember to meet with your doctor regarding your acid reflux concerns. Be prepared to talk about all of the options described here, so that you and your doctor can make an informed decision.

Finally, if you found this book useful in anyway, a review on Amazon is always appreciated!

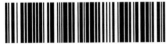

Made in the USA
Middletown, DE
09 September 2017